FORKS OVER KNIVES FOR BEGINNERS

Simple and Delicious Plant-Based Recipes for Better Wellness, Daily vitality and weight control.

By

LUNAR PUBLISHING

Writer name: Lunar Publishing

SEE MORE OF MY BOOKS

SCAN ME

Table of content

EXTRA

<28 Days Meal Planner>

Introduction

The Plant-Based Advantage

The introduction of this cookbook serves as a gateway to understanding the core principles and advantages of adopting a plant-based diet. It is the foundation upon which the entire book is built, setting the tone for the recipes and the overarching message of promoting health, managing weight, and achieving vitality through plant-based eating.

Plant-Based Eating Defined:

The introduction begins by defining what it means to follow a plant-based diet. It emphasizes that a plant-based diet is centered around whole, unprocessed plant foods. This includes fruits, vegetables, grains, legumes, nuts, and seeds while excluding or significantly reducing animal products such as meat, dairy, and eggs. The key idea is that the majority of your diet comes from plant sources.

Health Benefits:

One of the primary focuses of the introduction is to highlight the numerous health benefits associated with a plant-based diet. It discusses how this way of eating can reduce the risk of chronic diseases like heart disease, diabetes, and certain cancers. The author may delve into scientific research and studies that support these claims, illustrating that plant-based eating is not just a culinary preference but a well-documented path to better health.

Weight Management:

The introduction also touches on the concept of weight management. It explains how plant-based eating can be an effective strategy for achieving and maintaining a healthy weight. By choosing nutrient-dense, low-calorie foods, individuals can naturally manage their weight without counting calories or restricting portion sizes.

Vitality and Daily Wellness:

Vitality, or the state of being strong and active, is another key theme introduced in this section. The text discusses how a plant-based diet can boost energy levels, improve digestion, and enhance overall well-being. It may draw anecdotes or real-life examples of individuals who have experienced increased vitality after transitioning to a plant-based lifestyle.

The Purpose of the Cookbook:

The introduction sets clear expectations for the cookbook's purpose. It explains that the primary goal is to provide readers with a collection of 101 plant-based recipes that are not only nutritious but also delicious and easy to prepare. These recipes are intended to help readers incorporate more plant-based meals into their daily lives, regardless of their previous dietary habits.

A Call to Action:

Finally, the introduction often includes a call to action, encouraging readers to embark on a journey toward better health and vitality through plant-based eating. It may emphasize that this cookbook is not about strict diets or deprivation but about embracing a more wholesome and sustainable way of nourishing the body.

In essence, the introduction of "Forks Over Knives" serves as an informative and motivating prelude to the culinary adventure that follows in the subsequent chapters. It lays the groundwork for understanding the health benefits of a plant-based diet and sets the stage for readers to explore a variety of mouthwatering plant-based recipes designed to enhance their well-being and vitality.

Chapter 1: Energizing Breakfasts

Morning Sunshine Smoothie

Ingredients:
- 1 ripe banana
- 1 cup of fresh orange juice
- 1/2 cup of mango chunks (frozen or fresh)
- 1/2 cup of pineapple chunks (frozen or fresh)
- 1/2 cup of plain, unsweetened almond milk (or your preferred plant-based milk)
- 1 tablespoon of chia seeds (optional)
- 1 teaspoon of turmeric powder (optional)
- 1/2 cup of ice cubes (optional, for a colder smoothie)

Instructions:

1. **Prepare Your Ingredients:** Gather all your ingredients and make sure your fruits are appropriately prepared (e.g., peeled, chopped, and de-seeded if necessary).

2. **Start with the Base:** Begin by adding the ripe banana to your blender. Bananas provide natural sweetness and creaminess to the smoothie.

3. **Add the Citrus Zing:** Pour in the fresh orange juice. Oranges not only infuse a refreshing citrus flavor but also offer a dose of vitamin C.

4. **Tropical Vibes**: Include the mango chunks for a tropical twist. Mangoes add a luscious sweetness and a hint of tartness.

5. **Pineapple Paradise:** Add the pineapple chunks. Pineapples contribute to the smoothie's vibrant flavor with a tropical punch.

6. **Liquid Smoothness:** Pour in the almond milk (or your preferred plant-based milk). This helps to achieve the desired consistency and creaminess.

7. **Boost with Extras** (Optional): If you'd like to enhance the nutritional value, add chia seeds for fiber and omega-3 fatty acids, and a touch of turmeric for its potential anti-inflammatory properties.

8. **Chill It Down (Optional)**: If you prefer your smoothie cold, toss in some ice cubes for a refreshing chill.

9. **Blend to Perfection:** Secure the blender lid and blend all the ingredients until smooth. This usually takes around 30 seconds to 1 minute, depending on your blender's power.

10. **Taste Test:** Once blended, taste your Morning Sunshine Smoothie. Adjust the

sweetness or thickness by adding more fruit or almond milk if needed.

11. **Serve and Enjoy:** Pour the smoothie into a tall glass or a portable container if you're on the go. Garnish with a slice of orange or a sprinkle of chia seeds if desired.

This Morning Sunshine Smoothie is not only a burst of refreshing flavors but also a nourishing and energizing way to start your day. It provides essential vitamins, fiber, and hydration to kickstart your morning on the right note. Enjoy the vibrant and healthy beginning to your day!

Overnight Oats with Berries - Fueling Your Day Right

Ingredients:
- 1 cup of rolled oats
- 1 cup of your choice of plant-based milk (e.g., almond, soy, oat)
- 1/2 cup of mixed berries (e.g., strawberries, blueberries, raspberries)
- 1 tablespoon of maple syrup or agave nectar (adjust to taste)
- 1/2 teaspoon of vanilla extract
- A pinch of salt
- Optional toppings: Sliced bananas, chopped nuts, or additional berries

Instructions:

1. **Mix the Base**: In a container or mason jar, combine the rolled oats, plant-based milk, vanilla extract, maple syrup (or agave nectar), and a pinch of salt. Stir well to ensure the ingredients are evenly distributed.

15

2. **Layer with Berries**: Add half of your mixed berries on top of the oat mixture. This creates a delightful layer of fruity goodness.

3. **Repeat with Oats**: Add another layer of the oat mixture on top of the berries.

4. **Finish with Berries**: Top the oats with the remaining mixed berries. This will give your overnight oats a burst of color and flavor.

5. **Seal and Refrigerate:** Cover the container or jar and place it in the refrigerator. Let it sit overnight (or for at least 4 hours). This allows the oats to absorb the liquid and the flavors to meld.

6. **Serve and Customize:** In the morning, give your overnight oats a good stir. Feel free to add more plant-based milk if you prefer a thinner consistency. Top with sliced bananas, chopped nuts, or extra berries for added texture and flavor.

Avocado Toast with a Twist - Creamy and Nutrient-Packed

Ingredients:
- 2 slices of whole-grain or whole wheat bread (toasted)
- 1 ripe avocado
- 1 small tomato (sliced)
- 1/2 red onion (thinly sliced)
- A handful of fresh spinach leaves
- Salt and black pepper to taste
- A drizzle of olive oil (optional)

Instructions:

1. **Prepare the Avocado**: Cut the ripe avocado in half, remove the pit, and scoop out the flesh into a bowl. Mash it with a fork until it reaches your desired level of creaminess. Add a pinch of salt and black pepper to taste.

2. **Toast the Bread**: Toast your whole-grain or whole wheat bread slices until they are crispy and golden brown.

3. **Assemble the Toasts**: Spread the mashed avocado generously onto each slice of toast.

4. **Layer with Goodness**: Top the avocado with fresh spinach leaves, sliced tomatoes, and thinly sliced red onions. You can also drizzle a bit of olive oil for added flavor if desired.

5. **Season and Serve:** Season your avocado toast with a bit more salt and black pepper to taste. Serve immediately.

This Avocado Toast with a Twist is a delightful and nutrient-packed breakfast that combines the creamy goodness of avocado with the freshness of tomatoes and spinach. It's a simple yet satisfying way to start your day right, providing healthy fats, fiber, and vitamins. Enjoy this breakfast with a twist!

Chapter 2

Kale and Quinoa Salad

Ingredients:
- 1 cup quinoa, rinsed and drained
- 2 cups water or vegetable broth
- 1 bunch kale, stems removed and leaves thinly sliced
- 1 cup cherry tomatoes, halved
- 1/2 cucumber, diced
- 1/4 cup red onion, finely chopped
- 1/4 cup fresh parsley, chopped
- 1/4 cup extra-virgin olive oil
- 2 tablespoons lemon juice
- 1 clove garlic, minced
- Salt and pepper to taste
- Optional: 1/4 cup toasted pine nuts or slivered almonds for added crunch

Instructions:

1. **Prepare Quinoa**: In a medium saucepan, combine the quinoa and water or vegetable broth. Bring to a boil, then reduce the heat, cover, and simmer for about 15-20 minutes, or until the quinoa is cooked and the liquid is absorbed. Remove from heat and let it cool.

2. **Massage the Kale:** While the quinoa is cooking, place the thinly sliced kale in a large mixing bowl. Drizzle a bit of olive oil over the kale, add a pinch of salt, and massage the kale with your hands. This helps to tenderize the kale leaves and improve their texture.

3. **Prepare the Dressing:** In a small bowl, whisk together the remaining olive oil, lemon juice, minced garlic, salt, and pepper. This will be your zesty dressing for the salad.

4. **Assemble the Salad:** Once the quinoa has cooled, fluff it with a fork and add it to the bowl

with the kale. Toss in the halved cherry tomatoes, diced cucumber, finely chopped red onion, and fresh parsley.

5. **Drizzle and Toss:** Pour the prepared dressing over the salad ingredients. Gently toss everything together to ensure the dressing coats all the ingredients evenly.

6. **Optional Crunch:** If you desire some added crunch, sprinkle toasted pine nuts or slivered almonds on top.

7. **Serve and Enjoy:** Divide the salad into serving bowls, and it's ready to serve. This vibrant Kale and Quinoa Salad is not only packed with nutrients but bursting with flavors.

Notes:

- Feel free to customize this salad by adding your favorite vegetables or herbs.

- You can make the salad ahead of time, but add the dressing just before serving to keep it fresh and crisp.

This Kale and Quinoa Salad is a perfect representation of the chapter's theme, showcasing the use of wholesome, plant-based ingredients to create a nutritious and satisfying meal. It's a balanced combination of quinoa's protein and kale's nutrients, and the zesty dressing ties everything together for a delicious and healthy dining experience.

Tomato Basil Gazpacho: Summer in a Spoon

Ingredients:
- 6 ripe tomatoes, diced
- 1 cucumber, peeled, seeded, and diced
- 1 red bell pepper, diced
- 1/4 red onion, finely chopped
- 2 cloves garlic, minced
- 3 cups tomato juice
- 1/4 cup red wine vinegar
- 1/4 cup extra-virgin olive oil
- 1/4 cup fresh basil leaves, chopped
- Salt and pepper to taste

Instructions:

1. **Preparation**: In a large bowl, combine the diced tomatoes, cucumber, red bell pepper, finely chopped red onion, and minced garlic.

2. **Blending**: Transfer half of the vegetable mixture to a blender or food processor. Add 1.5 cups of tomato juice and blend until smooth. Pour the blended mixture into another large bowl.

3. **Texture**: Take the remaining vegetable mixture and pulse it briefly in the blender or food processor to achieve a chunkier texture. Add this to the smooth mixture in the large bowl.

4. **Flavor**: Stir in the red wine vinegar, extra-virgin olive oil, and fresh basil leaves. Season with salt and pepper to taste.

5. **Chill and Serve:** Cover the bowl and refrigerate the gazpacho for at least 2 hours or until well-chilled. This soup is meant to be served cold, making it a refreshing summer treat.

6. **Presentation**: Garnish with additional basil leaves before serving. Enjoy the taste of summer with this Tomato Basil Gazpacho!

Notes:

- Gazpacho can be customized with your favorite herbs or additional vegetables for added flavor and texture.

Miso Soup with Greens: A Warm Hug in a Bowl

Ingredients:
- 4 cups vegetable broth
- 1/4 cup miso paste (white or red, based on your preference)
- 1 cup sliced mushrooms (shiitake or button)
- 1 cup baby spinach or other greens of choice
- 2 green onions, thinly sliced
- 1 sheet nori (seaweed), cut into strips
- 1/2 cup tofu, cubed
- 1 teaspoon sesame oil (optional)
- Soy sauce or tamari to taste
- Sriracha or chili sauce (optional, for heat)

Instructions:

1. **Heat the Broth:** In a large pot, bring the vegetable broth to a simmer over medium heat.

2. **Dissolve the Miso**: In a small bowl, dissolve the miso paste in a ladleful of hot broth until it forms a smooth mixture. Then, add this back to the pot of broth.

3. **Mushrooms and Tofu:** Add the sliced mushrooms and cubed tofu to the pot. Simmer for about 5 minutes until the mushrooms are tender and the tofu is heated through.

4. **Greens and Nori:** Stir in the baby spinach or greens, sliced green onions, and nori strips. Cook for an additional 2-3 minutes until the greens wilt.

5. **Seasoning**: Add soy sauce or tamari to taste. If you like a bit of heat, you can also add Sriracha or chili sauce.

6. **Serve and Enjoy**: Ladle the warm miso soup into bowls, and optionally drizzle with a touch of sesame oil for extra flavor. This soup is like a

warm hug in a bowl, perfect for comfort and nourishment.

Notes:

- **Adjust the miso and soy sauce to your preferred saltiness level.**

- **Customize with your favorite veggies or additional seasonings to suit your taste.**

These two recipes from Chapter 2 of "Forks Over Knives" showcase the diversity of plant-based ingredients and flavors. The Tomato Basil Gazpacho is a refreshing and chilled soup perfect for hot summer days, while the Miso Soup with Greens provides warmth and comfort on cooler evenings, making them delightful additions to your plant-based culinary repertoire.

Chapter 3

Satisfying Sandwiches and Wraps

In this chapter, we'll explore three delightful and nutritious sandwich and wrap recipes that are not only easy to prepare but also perfect for satisfying your midday hunger. These recipes focus on incorporating plant-based ingredients that provide essential nutrients, flavor, and a satisfying crunch.

Hummus and Veggie Wrap: A Crunchy Delight

Ingredients:
- 1 large whole-grain or spinach tortilla wrap
- 2-3 tablespoons of your favorite hummus
- 1 cup of mixed salad greens (lettuce, spinach, arugula, etc.)
- 1/2 cup shredded carrots
- 1/2 cucumber, thinly sliced
- 1/2 red bell pepper, thinly sliced
- 1/4 red onion, thinly sliced
- Salt and pepper to taste
- Optional: Sprinkle of sunflower seeds or pumpkin seeds

Instructions:
1. Lay out the tortilla wrap on a clean surface, such as a cutting board or plate.

2. Spread a generous layer of hummus evenly over the entire surface of the tortilla, leaving a small border around the edges.

3. Place the mixed salad greens in the center of the tortilla, forming a horizontal line.

4. Add the shredded carrots, cucumber slices, red bell pepper slices, and red onion slices on top of the greens.

5. Season the veggies with a pinch of salt and pepper to taste.

6. If desired, sprinkle sunflower seeds or pumpkin seeds over the vegetables for added crunch and nutrition.

7. Carefully fold in the sides of the tortilla and then roll it up tightly from the bottom, creating a secure wrap.

8. Slice the wrap in half diagonally for easier handling or leave it whole for a more substantial meal.

9. Serve immediately, or wrap it in parchment paper or foil for an on-the-go lunch option.

Portobello Mushroom Burger: A Hearty Bite

Ingredients:
- 2 large Portobello mushroom caps
- 2 whole-grain burger buns
- 1/4 cup balsamic vinegar
- 2 cloves garlic, minced
- 2 tablespoons olive oil
- Salt and pepper to taste
- Your choice of burger toppings (lettuce, tomato, onion, avocado, etc.)

Instructions:

1. Clean the Portobello mushroom caps and remove the stems.

2. In a small bowl, whisk together the balsamic vinegar, minced garlic, olive oil, salt, and pepper to create a marinade.

3. Place the mushroom caps in a shallow dish and pour the marinade over them. Allow them to

marinate for at least 15-20 minutes, flipping them occasionally.

4. Preheat a grill or grill pan over medium-high heat.

5. Grill the marinated mushroom caps for about 4-5 minutes on each side, or until they are tender and have grill marks.

6. Toast the whole-grain burger buns on the grill for a minute or two until they are lightly browned.

7. Assemble your Portobello mushroom burgers with your choice of toppings on the toasted buns.

8. Serve hot, and enjoy the hearty, umami-rich flavor of these mushroom burgers.

Chickpea Salad Sandwich: A Protein-Packed Lunch

Ingredients:
- 1 can (15 ounces) of chickpeas (garbanzo beans), drained and rinsed
- 2 tablespoons vegan mayonnaise
- 1 tablespoon Dijon mustard
- 1/4 cup finely chopped celery
- 1/4 cup finely chopped red onion
- 1/4 cup pickle relish
- Salt and pepper to taste
- Lettuce leaves and whole-grain bread for serving

Instructions:
1. In a large bowl, mash the chickpeas with a fork or potato masher until they are mostly broken down but still slightly chunky.

2. Add the vegan mayonnaise, Dijon mustard, chopped celery, chopped red onion, and pickle relish to the mashed chickpeas.

3. Stir the ingredients together until they are well combined.

4. Season the chickpea salad with salt and pepper to taste. Adjust the seasoning to your preference.

5. To assemble the sandwiches, place lettuce leaves on a slice of whole-grain bread.

6. Spoon a generous portion of the chickpea salad onto the lettuce.

7. Top with another slice of whole-grain bread to complete the sandwich.

8. Optionally, you can add additional toppings like tomato slices or avocado.

9. Serve your protein-packed chickpea salad sandwich with a side of fresh veggies or a pickle spear.

These sandwich and wrap recipes in Chapter 3 offer a range of flavors and textures to satisfy your cravings while keeping your meal plant-based and nutritious. Whether you choose the crunchy Hummus and Veggie Wrap, the hearty Portobello Mushroom Burger, or the protein-packed Chickpea Salad Sandwich, you'll find these options both delicious and satisfying for your lunchtime needs.

Chapter 4: Delectable Dinner Creations

Lentil and Vegetable Stir-Fry: Quick and Flavorful

Ingredients:

- 1 cup of green or brown lentils, cooked and drained

- 2 cups of mixed vegetables (such as bell peppers, broccoli, and carrots), chopped

- 3 cloves of garlic, minced

- 1 tablespoon of fresh ginger, grated

- 2 tablespoons of low-sodium soy sauce or tamari

- 1 tablespoon of sesame oil (optional)

- 2 tablespoons of vegetable broth or water

- Salt and pepper to taste

- Sliced green onions and sesame seeds for garnish (optional)

Instructions:

1. Prepare the Lentils: Cook the lentils according to package instructions until they are tender. Drain and set aside.

2. Sauté Garlic and Ginger: In a large skillet or wok, heat a small amount of vegetable broth or water over medium-high heat. Add minced garlic and grated ginger, and sauté for about 1-2 minutes until fragrant.

3. Add Vegetables: Add the chopped mixed vegetables to the skillet. Stir-fry them for about

5-7 minutes until they begin to soften but are still crisp.

4. Combine Lentils: Add the cooked lentils to the skillet with the vegetables. Stir well to combine.

5. Soy Sauce and Seasoning: Drizzle the low-sodium soy sauce (or tamari) over the mixture and add sesame oil if desired. Stir to evenly coat the ingredients. Season with salt and pepper to taste.

6. Finish and Serve: Continue cooking for an additional 2-3 minutes, allowing the flavors to meld. Garnish with sliced green onions and sesame seeds if desired.

Butternut Squash Risotto: Creamy Comfort

Ingredients:

- 2 cups of butternut squash, diced
- 1 ½ cups of Arborio rice
- 4 cups of vegetable broth, heated
- 1 small onion, finely chopped
- 2 cloves of garlic, minced
- ½ cup of dry white wine (optional)
- 2 tablespoons of nutritional yeast (optional, for a cheesy flavor)
- Salt and black pepper to taste
- Fresh thyme leaves for garnish (optional)

Instructions:

1. **Roast the Butternut Squash**: Preheat your oven to 400°F (200°C). Place the diced butternut squash on a baking sheet, drizzle with olive oil,

and season with salt and pepper. Roast for about 25-30 minutes or until tender.

2. **Sauté Onion and Garlic**: In a large saucepan, heat a small amount of vegetable broth over medium heat. Add the chopped onion and minced garlic. Sauté until the onion becomes translucent, about 3-4 minutes.

3. **Add Arborio Rice:** Stir in the Arborio rice and cook for another 2 minutes until it becomes slightly translucent.

4. **Deglaze with Wine:** If using, pour in the dry white wine and stir until most of the liquid has been absorbed.

5. **Add Broth**: Begin adding the heated vegetable broth, one ladle at a time, stirring continuously. Allow the liquid to be absorbed before adding more. Continue this process until the rice is creamy and cooked to your desired consistency (usually about 18-20 minutes).

6. **Incorporate Butternut Squash**: Stir in the roasted butternut squash and nutritional yeast (if desired) during the last few minutes of cooking. Season with salt and black pepper to taste.

7. **Garnish and Serve:** Serve the risotto hot, garnished with fresh thyme leaves if desired.

Sweet Potato and Black Bean Enchiladas: A Spicy Fiesta

Ingredients:

- 2 large sweet potatoes, peeled and diced
- 1 can (15 oz) of black beans, drained and rinsed
- 1 red onion, finely chopped
- 1 red bell pepper, chopped
- 1 teaspoon of chili powder
- 1 teaspoon of ground cumin
- 1 teaspoon of smoked paprika
- 1 cup of enchilada sauce (store-bought or homemade)
- 8 whole wheat tortillas
- 1 cup of vegan shredded cheese (optional)
- Fresh cilantro leaves for garnish (optional)

Instructions:

1. **Roast Sweet Potatoes**: Preheat your oven to 400°F (200°C). Toss the diced sweet potatoes in olive oil and spread them on a baking sheet. Roast for about 20-25 minutes or until they are tender.

2. **Prepare Filling**: In a large skillet, sauté the chopped red onion and red bell pepper until they become tender. Add the chili powder, ground cumin, and smoked paprika. Stir in the black beans and roasted sweet potatoes. Cook for a few minutes to blend the flavors.

3. **Assemble Enchiladas:** Warm the whole wheat tortillas slightly. Place a portion of the sweet potato and black bean mixture in each tortilla, roll them up, and place them seam-side down in a baking dish.

4. **Pour Enchilada Sauce:** Pour the enchilada sauce over the rolled tortillas. If desired, sprinkle vegan shredded cheese on top.

5. **Bake**: Bake in the preheated oven at 350°F (175°C) for about 20 minutes or until the enchiladas are heated through, and the cheese (if used) is melted and bubbly.

6. **Garnish and Serve:** Garnish with fresh cilantro leaves if desired and serve hot.

These three recipes from Chapter 4 of "Forks Over Knives" offer a variety of flavors and textures. The Lentil and Vegetable Stir-Fry is a quick and nutritious option, the Butternut Squash Risotto provides creamy comfort with a touch of elegance, and the Sweet Potato and Black Bean Enchiladas bring a spicy fiesta to your plate. Enjoy these plant-based creations for a satisfying dinner experience that aligns with your wellness goals.

Chapter 5: Flavorful Sides and Snacks

Roasted Garlic Cauliflower: A Garlic Lover's Dream

Ingredients:
- 1 medium cauliflower head, cut into florets
- 4 cloves garlic, minced
- 2 tablespoons olive oil
- 1 teaspoon paprika
- 1/2 teaspoon salt
- 1/4 teaspoon black pepper
- 1 lemon, zested and juiced
- 2 tablespoons fresh parsley, chopped (for garnish)

Instructions:
1. Preheat your oven to 425°F (220°C).

2. In a large bowl, combine the cauliflower florets, minced garlic, olive oil, paprika, salt, and

black pepper. Toss everything together to ensure the cauliflower is evenly coated.

3. Spread the cauliflower mixture onto a baking sheet lined with parchment paper or a silicone baking mat.

4. Roast in the preheated oven for 20-25 minutes or until the cauliflower is tender and starts to brown at the edges.

5. While still hot, transfer the roasted cauliflower to a serving dish and drizzle with lemon juice and zest.

6. Garnish with fresh parsley.

7. Serve immediately as a flavorful side dish.

Notes:

- The roasting process caramelizes the cauliflower and enhances its natural sweetness, while the garlic adds a rich, savory flavor.

- The lemon zest and juice provide a bright and refreshing contrast to the roasted garlic.

Spiced Chickpea Snack: Crunchy and Irresistible

Ingredients:
- 2 cans (15 ounces each) chickpeas, drained and rinsed
- 2 tablespoons olive oil
- 1 teaspoon ground cumin
- 1/2 teaspoon smoked paprika
- 1/4 teaspoon cayenne pepper (adjust to taste)
- Salt to taste

Instructions:
1. Preheat your oven to 400°F (200°C).

2. In a large bowl, toss the drained chickpeas with olive oil, ground cumin, smoked paprika, cayenne pepper, and salt until evenly coated.

3. Spread the chickpeas on a baking sheet in a single layer.

4. Roast in the preheated oven for 20-25 minutes, or until the chickpeas are crispy and golden brown.

5. Let them cool slightly before serving as a crunchy snack.

Notes:

- This spiced chickpea snack is not only delicious but also high in protein and fiber, making it a healthy and satisfying snack option.

Quinoa-Stuffed Bell Peppers: Colorful and Nutrient-Rich

Ingredients:
- 4 large bell peppers, any color
- 1 cup quinoa, rinsed
- 2 cups vegetable broth
- 1 can (15 ounces) black beans, drained and rinsed
- 1 cup corn kernels (fresh or frozen)
- 1 cup diced tomatoes
- 1 teaspoon cumin
- 1/2 teaspoon chili powder
- Salt and pepper to taste
- 1 cup tomato sauce (for topping)
- Fresh cilantro leaves (for garnish)

Instructions:
1. Preheat your oven to 375°F (190°C).

2. Cut the tops off the bell peppers and remove the seeds and membranes.

3. In a saucepan, combine the quinoa and vegetable broth. Bring to a boil, then reduce heat, cover, and simmer for 15 minutes or until the quinoa is cooked and the liquid is absorbed.

4. In a large bowl, mix the cooked quinoa, black beans, corn, diced tomatoes, cumin, chili powder, salt, and pepper.

5. Stuff the bell peppers with the quinoa mixture and place them in a baking dish.

6. Pour tomato sauce over the stuffed peppers.

7. Cover the baking dish with foil and bake in the preheated oven for 25-30 minutes, or until the peppers are tender.

8. Garnish with fresh cilantro before serving.

Notes:

- These quinoa-stuffed bell peppers are not only visually appealing but also a nutritious and filling dish. The combination of quinoa, black beans, and vegetables provides a balanced meal.

These recipes from Chapter 5 of the cookbook offer a variety of flavors and textures, catering to different tastes and dietary preferences. Whether you're a garlic enthusiast, a lover of spicy snacks, or looking for a colorful and nutrient-rich main dish, this chapter has something for everyone. Enjoy the culinary journey and the health benefits these recipes bring to your table!

Chapter 6: Dessert of Desserts

Chocolate Avocado Mousse: Silky and Guilt-Free

Ingredients:
- 2 ripe avocados
- 1/4 cup unsweetened cocoa powder
- 1/4 cup maple syrup or agave nectar
- 1 tsp vanilla extract
- A pinch of salt
- 1/4 cup almond milk (or your preferred plant-based milk)
- Fresh berries and mint leaves for garnish (optional)

Instructions:
1. Scoop the flesh of the ripe avocados into a blender or food processor.

2. Add the unsweetened cocoa powder, maple syrup (or agave nectar), vanilla extract, and a pinch of salt to the blender.

3. Pour in the almond milk to help with blending.

4. Blend the mixture until it's completely smooth and has a silky texture. You may need to scrape down the sides of the blender and blend again to ensure everything is well combined.

5. Taste the mousse and adjust the sweetness if needed by adding more maple syrup.

6. Once the mousse is smooth and sweetened to your liking, transfer it to serving dishes or glasses.

7. Chill the mousse in the refrigerator for at least 30 minutes to let it set.

8. Before serving, garnish with fresh berries and mint leaves for a pop of color and freshness.

Berry Bliss Parfait: Layers of Sweetness

Ingredients:
- 2 cups of mixed berries (strawberries, blueberries, raspberries)
- 1 cup of dairy-free yogurt (e.g., almond or coconut yogurt)
- 1/2 cup of granola (look for a plant-based option)
- 1 tbsp maple syrup (optional, for added sweetness)
- Fresh mint leaves for garnish (optional)

Instructions:
1. Wash and prepare the mixed berries. You can slice the strawberries and leave the other berries whole.

2. In a bowl, mix the dairy-free yogurt with maple syrup if you prefer it sweeter.

3. Start assembling the parfait in glasses or bowls. Begin with a layer of yogurt at the bottom.

4. Add a layer of granola on top of the yogurt.

5. Add a layer of mixed berries.

6. Repeat the layers until you've used up all the ingredients or reached your desired serving size.

7. Finish with a few fresh mint leaves for garnish.

Banana Walnut Pancakes: Breakfast for Dessert

Ingredients:
- 2 ripe bananas
- 1 cup of whole wheat flour (or gluten-free flour if preferred)
- 1 tsp baking powder
- 1/2 tsp ground cinnamon
- 1/4 cup chopped walnuts
- 1 cup plant-based milk (e.g., almond, soy, or oat milk)
- 1 tsp vanilla extract
- Maple syrup for drizzling
- Sliced bananas and extra chopped walnuts for topping

Instructions:
1. In a mixing bowl, mash the ripe bananas until smooth.

2. Add the whole wheat flour, baking powder, ground cinnamon, and chopped walnuts to the mashed bananas.

3. Pour in the plant-based milk and vanilla extract.

4. Stir the mixture until all the ingredients are well combined.

5. Heat a non-stick skillet or griddle over medium heat and lightly grease it.

6. Pour ladlefuls of the pancake batter onto the skillet to form pancakes.

7. Cook until bubbles form on the surface, then flip and cook the other side until golden brown.

8. Serve the pancakes hot, drizzled with maple syrup, and topped with sliced bananas and extra chopped walnuts.

These dessert recipes in Chapter 6 offer a range of sweet treats that are not only delicious but also guilt-free, using plant-based ingredients to create delightful flavors. Enjoy the silky Chocolate Avocado Mousse, the refreshing Berry Bliss Parfait, and the indulgent Banana Walnut Pancakes that can even be enjoyed as a dessert!

Chapter 7

Green Goodness Smoothie: A Sip of Health

Ingredients:
- 1 cup fresh spinach leaves
- 1/2 cucumber, peeled and sliced
- 1 ripe banana
- 1/2 cup pineapple chunks
- 1/2 cup unsweetened almond milk (or your preferred plant-based milk)
- 1 tablespoon chia seeds
- 1 teaspoon honey (optional, for added sweetness)
- Ice cubes (optional, for a colder smoothie)

Instructions:

1. Start by washing the fresh spinach leaves thoroughly and then placing them in a blender.

2. Add the peeled and sliced cucumber, ripe banana, pineapple chunks, and chia seeds to the blender.

3. Pour in the unsweetened almond milk (or your chosen plant-based milk) to help with blending. If you prefer a sweeter smoothie, you can add a teaspoon of honey at this stage.

4. If you like your smoothie extra chilly, toss in a few ice cubes as well.

5. Blend all the ingredients until you achieve a smooth and creamy consistency.

6. Once blended, pour your Green Goodness Smoothie into a glass, and it's ready to enjoy! This vibrant green concoction is packed with nutrients and is a refreshing way to start your day or refuel after a workout.

Turmeric Golden Milk: Anti-Inflammatory Elixir

Ingredients:
- 1 cup unsweetened almond milk (or your preferred plant-based milk)
- 1/2 teaspoon ground turmeric
- 1/4 teaspoon ground cinnamon
- A pinch of black pepper (enhances turmeric absorption)
- 1 teaspoon honey (or maple syrup for a vegan option)

Instructions:

1. In a small saucepan, heat the unsweetened almond milk over low to medium heat.

2. As the milk begins to warm, add the ground turmeric and ground cinnamon. Whisk them gently into the milk.

3. Add a pinch of black pepper to enhance the absorption of turmeric's beneficial properties.

4. Continue to heat the mixture, stirring frequently, until it's hot but not boiling.

5. Remove the saucepan from the heat and let it cool slightly.

6. Sweeten your Turmeric Golden Milk with honey or maple syrup, adjusting the sweetness to your preference.

7. Pour your elixir into a mug, and it's ready to sip! Turmeric Golden Milk is known for its anti-inflammatory properties and soothing qualities, making it a perfect beverage to unwind with.

Refreshing Cucumber Mint Cooler: A Summer Chill

Ingredients:
- 1 cucumber, sliced
- Juice of 2 fresh lemons
- A handful of fresh mint leaves
- 2 tablespoons honey (or agave syrup for a vegan option)
- Ice cubes

Instructions:

1. Place the sliced cucumber, fresh lemon juice, and fresh mint leaves in a blender.

2. Add the honey (or agave syrup) for a touch of sweetness.

3. If you prefer a colder drink, add some ice cubes to the blender.

4. Blend all the ingredients until smooth.

5. Pour your Refreshing Cucumber Mint Cooler into glasses filled with ice cubes.

6. Garnish with extra mint leaves or a lemon slice if desired.

7. Sip and savor the refreshing flavors of this summer cooler, perfect for staying hydrated on hot days. The combination of cucumber and mint provides a delightful burst of coolness, while the lemon adds a zesty twist.

These three recipes from Chapter 7 offer a variety of flavors and health benefits. The Green Goodness Smoothie is a nutrient-packed morning boost, Turmeric Golden Milk is a soothing elixir with anti-inflammatory properties, and the Refreshing Cucumber Mint Cooler is a delightful and hydrating summer refreshment. Enjoy these delicious and healthful drinks as part of your plant-based culinary journey.

Chapter 8

Holiday Stuffed Squash: Festive and Flavorful

This chapter is all about bringing a touch of elegance and festivity to your holiday table with a delightful recipe for Holiday Stuffed Squash. This dish is not only visually appealing but also packed with the flavors of the season. It's perfect for Thanksgiving, Christmas, or any special occasion when you want to impress your guests with a plant-based centerpiece.

Ingredients for Holiday Stuffed Squash:

- 4 acorn or carnival squash
- 2 cups cooked quinoa
- 1 cup chopped kale
- 1 cup dried cranberries
- 1 cup chopped pecans
- 1/2 cup diced red onion
- 2 cloves garlic, minced
- 2 tablespoons olive oil
- 2 teaspoons fresh thyme leaves
- Salt and pepper to taste
- Maple syrup for drizzling (optional)

Instructions for Holiday Stuffed Squash:

1. **Prepare the Squash:**
   - Preheat your oven to 375°F (190°C).

   - Slice the tops off the squash and scoop out the seeds.

- Brush the inside of the squash with olive oil and sprinkle with salt and pepper.

- Place the squash, cut side down, on a baking sheet.

- Bake for about 30-40 minutes, or until the squash is tender.

2. Prepare the Filling:

- While the squash is baking, heat 2 tablespoons of olive oil in a large skillet over medium heat.

- Add the diced red onion and minced garlic. Sauté until fragrant and translucent.

- Stir in the chopped kale and cook until it wilts.

- Add the cooked quinoa, dried cranberries, chopped pecans, and fresh thyme leaves to the skillet. Mix well.

- Season with salt and pepper to taste. Cook for an additional 5 minutes, allowing the flavors to meld.

3. **Stuff the Squash**:

- Once the squash is tender, remove it from the oven.

- Carefully flip the squash over and stuff each cavity with the quinoa mixture.

- Place the stuffed squash back in the oven and bake for an additional 15-20 minutes, or until the filling is heated through and the tops are slightly crispy.

4. **Serve and Drizzle (Optional):**

- Remove the stuffed squash from the oven and let them cool slightly.

- Before serving, you can drizzle a touch of maple syrup over the top for a hint of sweetness and extra holiday flair.

Mouthwatering Veggie Lasagna: Layers of Celebration

This section takes you on a culinary journey through a hearty and indulgent Veggie Lasagna. It's a dish that showcases layers of colorful vegetables, rich tomato sauce, and creamy plant-based béchamel sauce. This mouthwatering lasagna is a celebration of flavors and textures, perfect for gatherings or special occasions.

Ingredients for Mouthwatering Veggie Lasagna:
- 12 lasagna noodles, cooked al dente
- 2 cups marinara sauce
- 2 cups spinach, chopped
- 2 cups sliced mushrooms
- 1 cup diced red bell pepper
- 1 cup diced zucchini
- 1 cup diced yellow squash
- 1 cup diced onion
- 2 cloves garlic, minced

- 2 cups plant-based béchamel sauce (made with almond milk)
- 1 cup vegan mozzarella cheese
- Salt and pepper to taste
- Fresh basil leaves for garnish (optional)

Instructions for Mouthwatering Veggie Lasagna:

1. **Prepare the Vegetables:**
   - In a large skillet, heat olive oil over medium heat.

   - Add diced onion and minced garlic. Sauté until fragrant and translucent.

   - Add mushrooms, red bell pepper, zucchini, and yellow squash. Cook until vegetables are tender. Season with salt and pepper.

2. **Assemble the Lasagna:**
   - Preheat your oven to 350°F (175°C).

- In a baking dish, spread a layer of marinara sauce on the bottom.

- Place a layer of cooked lasagna noodles over the sauce.

- Add a layer of sautéed vegetables, followed by a layer of chopped spinach.

- Pour a portion of plant-based béchamel sauce over the spinach.

- Repeat these layers until you've used all the ingredients, finishing with a layer of marinara sauce on top.

- Sprinkle vegan mozzarella cheese over the lasagna.

3. **Bake and Serve:**
- Cover the baking dish with foil and bake for 25-30 minutes, or until the lasagna is bubbling and the cheese is melted.

- Remove from the oven and let it cool slightly before serving.

- Garnish with fresh basil leaves if desired.

Plant-Based Thanksgiving: A Bountiful Spread

This section in Chapter 8 is a treasure trove of recipes designed to create a memorable and entirely plant-based Thanksgiving feast. Whether you're hosting a gathering or attending as a guest, these dishes will leave everyone at the table asking for seconds. Here are some of the recipes featured in this bountiful spread:

1. **Plant-Based Stuffing**: A hearty blend of bread, vegetables, herbs, and plant-based butter creates a stuffing that's rich in flavor and texture.

2. **Creamy Mashed Potatoes:** Creamy Yukon Gold or sweet potatoes mashed with plant-based milk and a hint of garlic result in velvety smooth goodness.

3. **Vegan Gravy**: A luscious gravy made from vegetable broth, flour, and savory seasonings to drizzle over potatoes and stuffing.

4. **Cranberry Orange Sauce:** Fresh cranberries simmered with orange zest and a touch of sweetness for a delightful, tangy side dish.

5. **Green Bean Almondine:** Crisp green beans sautéed with slivered almonds in plant-based butter for a perfect complement to the meal.

6. **Roasted Root Vegetables:** A medley of carrots, parsnips, and beets roasted to caramelized perfection with herbs and olive oil.

7. **Pumpkin Pie:** A spiced pumpkin filling in a flaky plant-based pie crust, topped with dairy-free whipped cream for dessert.

8. **Apple-Cranberry Crisp:** A warm and fruity dessert featuring apples and cranberries baked to a golden crisp, with a crunchy topping.

9. **Plant-Based Holiday Roast**: A centerpiece dish made from plant-based proteins like seitan or tempeh, marinated and roasted to perfection.

Each recipe in this Thanksgiving spread is carefully crafted to capture the essence of a traditional holiday meal while maintaining a plant-based approach. The ingredients and instructions for each dish ensure that you can create a festive, satisfying, and compassionate Thanksgiving dinner that will leave everyone grateful for the delicious flavors and the mindful choices made to protect the planet and your health.

So, whether you're celebrating Thanksgiving or any special occasion, the Plant-Based Thanksgiving spread in Chapter 8 of "Forks Over Knives" has you covered with recipes that embrace the joy of feasting while aligning with a plant-based lifestyle. Enjoy the bountiful flavors and the warmth of gathering with loved ones!

FORKS OVER KNIVES FOR BEGINNERS   SIMPLE AND DELICIOUS PLANT-BASED
RECIPES FOR BETTER WELLNESS, DAILY VITALITY AND WEIGHT CONTROL

Chapter 9

Weekly Meal Planner: Your Roadmap to Success

In this chapter, we'll dive into the practical aspects of incorporating a plant-based diet into your everyday life. The Weekly Meal Planner serves as your essential tool for organizing your meals, making grocery lists, and ensuring a balanced diet throughout the week.

Weekly Meal Planner: Your Roadmap to Success

Ingredients:

To successfully plan your plant-based meals, you'll need:

1. **Meal Planning Calendar**: This is your blank canvas for the week. Use it to map out breakfasts, lunches, dinners, and snacks for each day.

2. **Recipe Collection**: Gather all the recipes from previous chapters and list them in your planner.

3. **Grocery List:** Create a list of ingredients needed for the week based on your selected recipes.

4. **Post-It Notes or Sticky Tabs:** Use these to mark recipes you plan to prepare.

5. **Pens, Pencils, and Highlighters**: For jotting down notes, making adjustments, and highlighting important items.

Instructions:

1. **Select Your Recipes:** Start by browsing the recipes in this cookbook. Consider your dietary preferences, any dietary restrictions, and the ingredients you have on hand.

2. **Plan Your Meals**: Begin filling out your Meal Planning Calendar with recipes for each meal and snack. Be sure to balance your meals, incorporating a variety of flavors, ingredients, and cuisines throughout the week.

3. **Check Your Pantry**: Review your pantry and fridge for ingredients you already have. Mark them off on your grocery list.

4. **Create Your Grocery List:** Use the list of ingredients from your selected recipes to create a comprehensive grocery list. Organize it by category (e.g., produce, pantry staples, condiments) for easier shopping.

5. **Shop Mindfully:** When shopping for groceries, stick to your list to avoid unnecessary purchases. Look for fresh, seasonal produce and high-quality pantry staples.

6. **Prep in Advance**: If time allows, do some prep work in advance. Chop vegetables, cook grains, or make sauces that can be refrigerated until needed.

7. **Follow Your Plan:** Throughout the week, refer to your Meal Planning Calendar to guide your meal preparation. Stick to your plan as closely as possible, making adjustments as needed.

8. **Enjoy the Benefits:** A well-structured meal plan simplifies your plant-based journey,

reduces food waste, and ensures balanced nutrition. It also saves time and makes grocery shopping a breeze.

Stocking Your Plant-Based Pantry: Essentials for Every Kitchen

Ingredients:

Stocking your plant-based pantry requires having these essentials:

1. **Whole Grains:** Brown rice, quinoa, oats, and whole wheat pasta.

2. **Legumes**: Canned or dried beans (black beans, chickpeas, lentils).

3. **Nuts and Seeds:** Almonds, walnuts, chia seeds, and flaxseeds.

4. **Plant-Based Proteins:** Tofu, tempeh, and plant-based protein powders.

5. **Non-Dairy Milk:** Almond, soy, or oat milk.

6. **Herbs and Spices:** A variety of herbs, spices, and seasonings for flavor.

7. **Healthy Fats**: Olive oil, avocado oil, and nut butters.

8. **Canned Tomatoes**: Diced and crushed tomatoes for sauces.

9. **Condiments**: Soy sauce, tahini, and nutritional yeast.

10. **Sweeteners**: Maple syrup, agave nectar, or dates for natural sweetness.

Instructions:

1. **Assess Your Pantry:** Take inventory of what you already have and what needs replenishing.

2. **Organize Your Pantry:** Arrange your pantry items in a logical order, making them easy to access while cooking.

3. **Label and Date**: Label containers with purchase dates to ensure freshness.

4. **Rotate Stock:** Use older items before newer ones to reduce food waste.

5. **Regular Replenishment:** Make it a habit to restock pantry essentials regularly.

Eating Out the Plant-Based Way: Navigating Restaurants

Ingredients:

When dining out at restaurants, consider these ingredients:

1. **Menu Knowledge**: Familiarize yourself with the menu options available at the restaurant.

2. **Special Requests**: Be prepared to make special requests to accommodate your plant-based preferences.

3. **Substitutions:** Know which ingredients can be substituted or omitted to make dishes plant-based.

4. **Communication**: Communicate your dietary needs clearly and politely with the server.

5. **Patience**: Be patient with restaurant staff, as not all establishments may be accustomed to plant-based requests.

Instructions:

1. **Select Plant-Based Friendly Restaurants**: Choose restaurants that offer a variety of plant-based options or have a flexible menu.

2. **Menu Exploration:** Explore the menu thoroughly and inquire about ingredient lists for dishes.

3. **Customize Your Order:** Don't hesitate to customize dishes to suit your preferences. Ask for substitutions or removal of non-plant-based ingredients.

4. **Ask Questions**: If unsure, don't hesitate to ask your server about preparation methods and ingredients.

5. **Enjoy Your Meal**: With a little planning and communication, you can savor a delicious plant-based meal at a restaurant.

By following these guidelines in Chapter 8, you'll master the art of planning your plant-based meals, stocking your pantry with essentials, and confidently navigating restaurants to enjoy plant-based options even when dining out. These practical tips will enhance your plant-based lifestyle and make it more accessible and enjoyable.

Conclusion

Conclusion: Your Journey Towards Wellness

The conclusion of this cookbook is more than just the end of a culinary journey; it's a culmination of the principles, knowledge, and practical guidance that the book has offered to its readers.

1. **Reflection on Wellness:** In this section, the author reflects on the overarching theme of the book, which is promoting wellness through a plant-based diet. It reiterates the core message that the recipes provided throughout the book are not just about delicious meals; they are a path to better health, weight management, and overall vitality.

2. **Encouragement and Inspiration:** The conclusion serves as a source of motivation and encouragement for the readers. It acknowledges that transitioning to a plant-based diet can be a significant change for some, and it can come

with challenges. However, it emphasizes that the journey toward wellness is worth every effort. It reassures readers that even small steps towards incorporating plant-based meals into their diet can have a positive impact on their health.

3. **A Call to Action:** To ensure that readers continue on their path to wellness, the conclusion may contain a call to action. This could involve encouraging readers to set specific goals, create meal plans, or engage in ongoing education about plant-based nutrition. It may also suggest connecting with local or online communities of like-minded individuals for support and recipe sharing.

In summary, the conclusion of "Forks Over Knives" is a pivotal part of the book that not only marks the end of the recipe collection but also serves as a guidepost for readers as they continue their journey toward enhanced wellness, weight management, and daily vitality through plant-based eating. It encourages, inspires, and equips readers with the knowledge

and resources they need to embrace a healthier
and more vibrant lifestyle.

EXTRA

<28 Days Meal Planner>

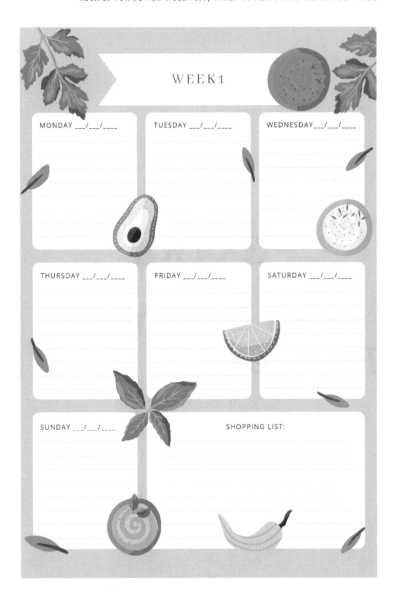

WEEK 1

MONDAY ___/___/____

TUESDAY ___/___/____

WEDNESDAY___/___/____

THURSDAY ___/___/____

FRIDAY ___/___/____

SATURDAY ___/___/____

SUNDAY ___/___/____

SHOPPING LIST:

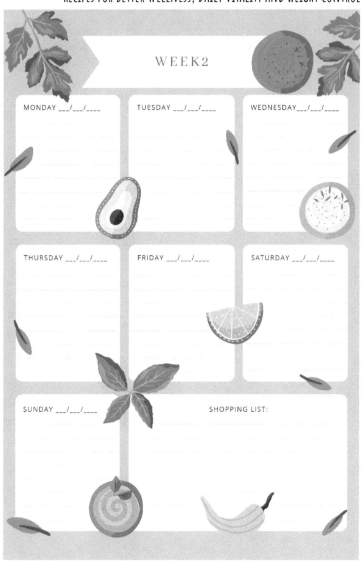

WEEK2

MONDAY ___/___/____

TUESDAY ___/___/____

WEDNESDAY___/___/____

THURSDAY ___/___/____

FRIDAY ___/___/____

SATURDAY ___/___/____

SUNDAY ___/___/____

SHOPPING LIST:

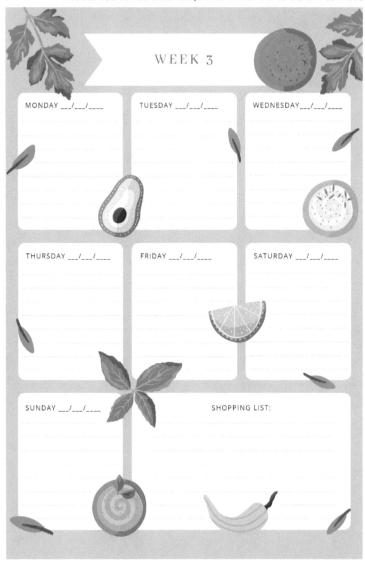

WEEK 3

MONDAY ___/___/____

TUESDAY ___/___/____

WEDNESDAY___/___/____

THURSDAY ___/___/____

FRIDAY ___/___/____

SATURDAY ___/___/____

SUNDAY ___/___/____

SHOPPING LIST: